"HOW TO DO KETO"

A complete guide to Keto diet and how to do keto the right way. A must read for all keto lovers for a healthier lifestyle and fulfilling your keto goals!

By Albert Millie Hawthorn

TABLE OF CONTENT

CHAPTER ONE

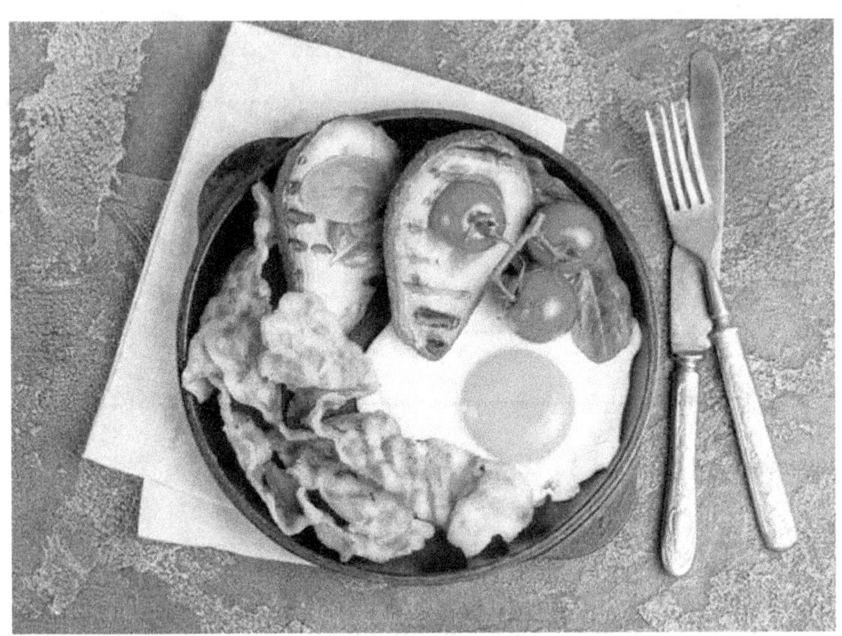

Understanding Keto Diet

The keto diet includes mainly fats, moderate protein and a small amount of carbohydrates. Eating a lot of fat and too little carbohydrate puts you in a ketosis, a metabolic state in which your body burns fat instead of carbs as fuel.

There are different types of keto diets, including the standard diet, keto keto and dirty keto. Keto works for many people, but it can also cause side effects such as fatigue and digestive problems.

What is Keto Diet?

The keto diet is an abbreviation for "ketogenic diet". It is a diet high in fat and low in carbohydrates that can turn your body into a machine to burn fat.

The keto diet changes the way your body converts food into energy. Normally, your body transforms carbohydrates (think of bread and pasta) into glucose into energy. Eating a lot of fat and too few carbohydrates puts you in ketosis, a metabolic state in which your body burns fat instead of carbohydrates as fuel.

What is Ketone?

When your body cannot absorb glucose from your diet, your liver converts fats in your diet into molecules called ketones, an alternative source of fuel. This puts it in ketosis, also known as premium weight loss mode.

You are in ketosis when your ketones reach 0.8 millimoles per liter. The keto diet is a way to make your body produce ketones. Other ways of working with ketones include intermittent fasting and the use of your glucose stores while exercising.

Advantages of Keto Diet

The keto diet rapidly increases weight loss because your body converts fat from your diet and fat stores into ketones. And unlike glucose, ketones cannot be stored as fats because they are not digested in the same way.

It is amazing, isn't it? For decades, you've heard that fat makes you fat. Your body is designed to use fats as an alternative source of fuel. For most of the story, people did not eat three meals and snacks during the day. Instead, humans should hunt and harvest their food and they learned to thrive when there was no food available, sometimes for days and days.

<u>HERE ARE JUST A FEW BENEFITS OF A KETOGENIC DIET:</u>

The application and implementation of the ketogenic diet has grown considerably. Ketogenic diets are often indicated in the treatment plan in a number of medical conditions.

Epilepsy: This is the main reason for the development of the ketogenic diet. For some reason, the rate of epileptic seizures is reduced when patients receive a keto diet.

The cases of pediatric epilepsy are the most sensitive to the keto diet. There are children who have experience in eliminating seizures after a few years of using a keto diet. In general, children with epilepsy need to fast a few days before starting the ketogenic diet as part of their treatment.

Cancer: Research suggests that the therapeutic efficacy of ketogenic diets against tumor growth can be improved when combined with certain drugs and procedures in a "heartbeat" paradigm.

It is also promising to note that ketogenic diets lead to remission of cancer cells. This means that keto diets "starve the cancer" to reduce the symptoms.

Alzheimer's disease: There are several indications that the memory functions of patients with Alzheimer's disease improve after a ketogenic diet.

Ketones are an excellent alternative energy source for the brain, especially when it has become insulin resistant. Ketones also provide substrates (cholesterol) that help repair damaged neurons and membranes. All of this helps improve memory and cognition in patients with Alzheimer's disease.

Diabetes: In general, it is accepted that carbohydrates are the main cause of diabetes. Therefore, by reducing the amount of carbohydrate ingested through a ketogenic diet, there is more chance of improving blood glucose control. In addition, the combination of a keto diet with other diabetes treatment plans can significantly improve your overall effectiveness.

Gluten allergy: Many people allergic to gluten are not diagnosed with this condition. However, monitoring a ketogenic diet has shown an improvement in associated symptoms, such as digestive discomfort and swelling.

Most carbohydrate foods are rich in gluten. Therefore, when using a keto diet, much of the gluten intake is minimized due to the elimination of a wide variety of carbohydrates.

CHAPTER TWO

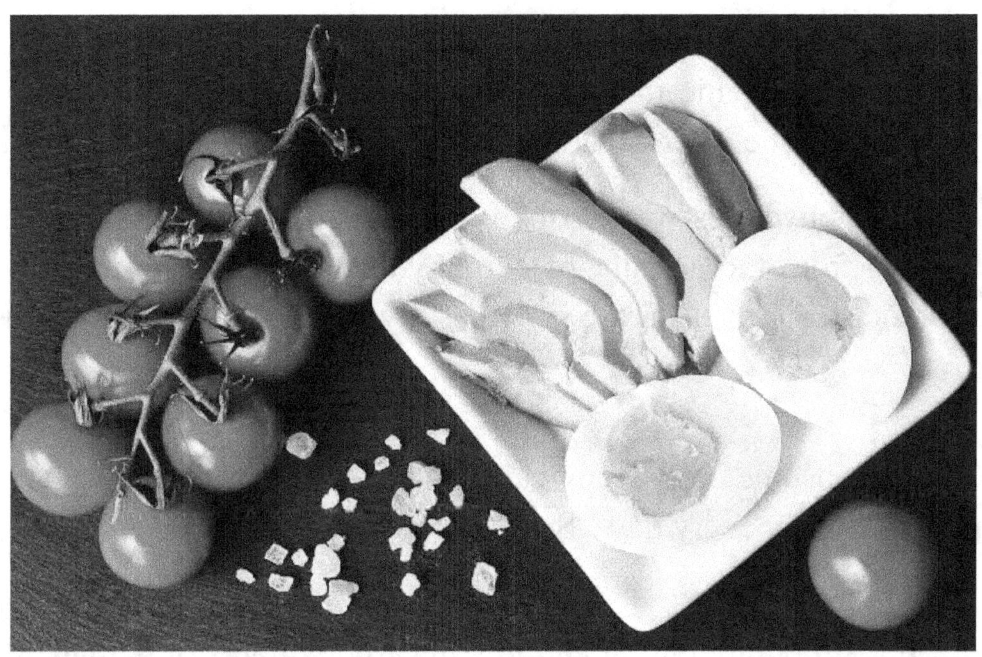

How Ketones affect your hormones

Ketones have an impact on cholecystokinin (CCK), a hormone that satisfies you, and on ghrelin, the "hunger hormone."

CCK: Your intestines are released from CCK after eating, which makes it a powerful regulator of food consumption, so much so that injecting CCK into people will stop them from eating. [9] Ketones increase CCK levels, so you are very happy after meals.

Ghrelin: Ghrelin is called "the hunger hormone" because it increases appetite. It is released from the stomach and intestines, and blood levels peak when you fast. When you finally eat a meal, ghrelin falls in response to the nutrients that circulate in your blood. Ketosis suppresses the increase in ghrelin levels associated with weight loss. [10] Therefore, when you have ketosis, you don't constantly think about your next meal.

What to eat in a keto diet

The keto diet is ⬜uite simple: eat mostly healthy fats (75% of your daily calories), protein (20%) and a very small amount of carbohydrates (5%). This combo will put you in nutritional ketosis.

Choose low carb foods like meat, fish, eggs, vegetables and good fats. Check out this detailed list of ketogenic foods and explore these keto recipes for meal ideas. Most people eat better between 30 and 150 grams of net carbohydrates a day.

The term "net carbohydrates" means that you can subtract fiber and sugar alcohols (such as xylitol) from the amount of carbohydrates you consume daily; do not affect your blood sugar levels or are stored as glycogen, the form of glucose stored

Types of keto diet

Standard keto: consume very few carbohydrates (less than 50 grams of net carbohydrates per day), every day. Some keto enthusiasts consume only 20 grams a day.

Cyclic keto: Eat a food high in fat and low in carbohydrates (less than 50 grams of net carbohydrates a day) five to six days a week. On the seventh day, have a carbohydrate diet day (approximately 150 grams). The bulletproof diet falls into this category, but modifies the keto for better performance with intermittent fasting, protein fasting and an emphasis on nutrient-rich and low-flammable foods. Download the free roadmap for an infallible scheme here.

Directed keto: follow the standard keto diet, but eat additional carbohydrates 30 minutes to an hour before high intensity training. Glucose is intended to improve performance and return to ketosis after training. If your energy suffers in the gym during the keto, this feeding style might work for you.

Dirty keto: the dirty keto follows the same proportion of fat, protein and carbohydrates as the usual keto diet, but by the way: regardless of the origin of these macronutrients. Dinner could be a Big Mac without bread with a Pepsi diet. Learn more about the dirty keto diet and how it works.

Moderate keto: Eat a lot of fat with 100 to 150 grams of net carbohydrates every day. Women often get better results with this diet: restrictive carbohydrates can sometimes affect hormonal function. In addition, some athletes discover that they burn with less than 100 grams of carbohydrates on training days.

How to find which approach works best for you

First, consult your doctor before making any major dietary changes.

Try different styles of keto for at least a month each.

Track your carbohydrates, fat and protein with a food tracking app like MyFitnessPal and My Macros +.

Set goals based on fat and carbohydrate intake instead of calories. Eat until you are full and listen to your body.

Are you more acute with a weekly carbohydrate balance or do you do better with a complete ketogenic diet? Do you burn when immersing less than 100 grams of carbohydrates a day? There is a lot of variation in low carbs, and some people feel better with different feeding styles. Find the right balance that best suits your personal biology.

Secondary effect of keto (and what to do about it)

In general, a ketogenic diet is perfectly safe for many people, but there are some side effects to consider:

Dehydration and muscle cramps

Carbohydrates need water to be stored. Fat no. In a keto diet, you store less water and your kidneys actively expel sodium instead of holding it back. That means it's easy to get dehydrated by eating keto, especially during the first few weeks. With dehydration and low electrolytes, your muscles may also begin to suffer from cramps.

Cramps caused by the keto diet

Do this: double magnesium, sodium and potassium, the three main electrolytes in your body, and make sure to drink more water. This is especially important if you exercise keto. Staying hydrated will also help you avoid the symptoms of keto flu (more details below).

Decrease in metabolic flexibility

Many people report having difficulty assimilating carbohydrates when following a strict keto diet in the long run, which makes sense. If you almost never eat carbohydrates, you do not need to keep your insulin pathways running smoothly. It's like keeping the light on during the day: a waste of energy.

Your body seems to reduce the regulation of insulin (the hormone that directs your cells to use carbohydrates as fuel) after being strictly keto for a while. Some parts of your body develop with glucose, such as the glial cells in your brain that manage repair and immune function. If your cells are excellent at using fat as fuel and bad for carbohydrates, they will not work at full power.

CHAPTER THREE

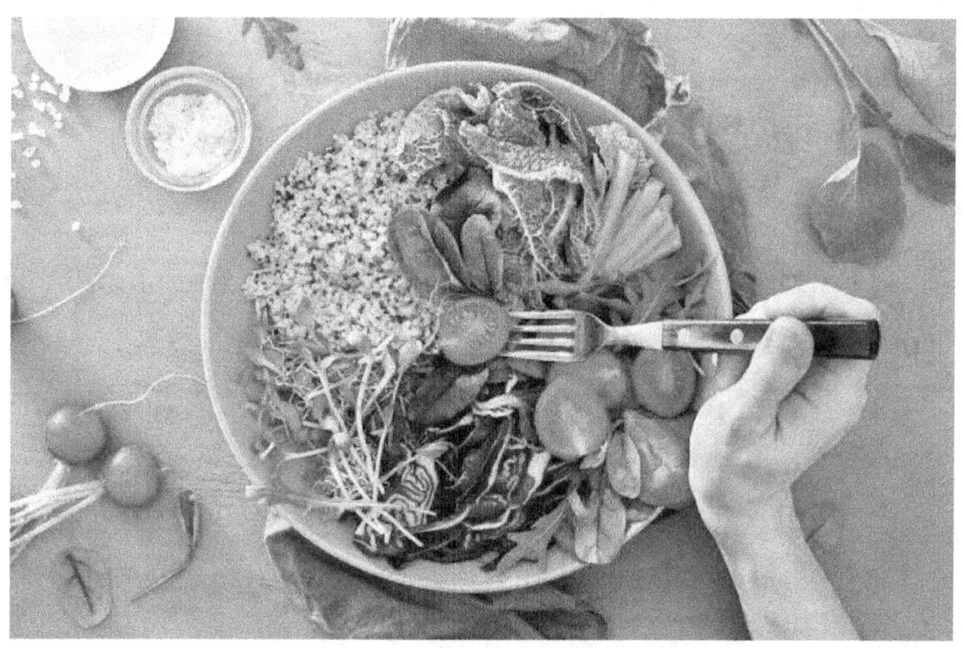

Keto Dieting? Here Are 10 Foods You Must Have In Your Kitchen

The ketogenic diet is a very successful weight-loss program. It utilizes high fat and low carbohydrate ingredients in order to burn fat instead of glucose. Many people are familiar with the Atkins diet, but the keto plan restricts carbs even more.

Because we are surrounded by fast food restaurants and processed meals, it can be a challenge to avoid carb-rich foods, but proper planning can help.

Plan menus and snacks at least a week ahead of time, so you aren't caught with only high carb meal choices. Research keto recipes online; there are quite a few good ones to choose from. Immerse yourself in the keto lifestyle, find your favorite recipes, and stick with them.

There are a few items that are staples of a keto diet. Be sure to have these items on hand:

Eggs - Used in omelets, quiches (yes, heavy cream is legal on keto!), hard boiled as a snack, low carb pizza crust, and more; if you like eggs, you have a great chance of success on this diet

Bacon - Do I need a reason? breakfast, salad garnish, burger topper, BLT's (no bread of course; try a BLT in a bowl, tossed in mayo)

Cream cheese - Dozens of recipes, pizza crusts, main dishes, desserts

Shredded cheese - Sprinkle over taco meat in a bowl, made into tortilla chips in the microwave, salad toppers, low-carb pizza and enchiladas

Lots of romaine and spinach - Fill up on the green veggies; have plenty on hand for a quick salad when hunger pangs hit

EZ-Sweetz liquid sweetener - Use a couple of drops in place of sugar; this artificial sweetener is the most natural and easiest to use that I've found

Cauliflower - Fresh or frozen bags you can eat this low-carb veggie by itself, tossed in olive oil and baked, mashed in fake potatoes, chopped/shredded and used in place of rice under main dishes, in low-carb and keto pizza crusts, and much more

Frozen chicken tenders - Have a large bag on hand; thaw quickly and grill, saute, mix with veggies and top with garlic sauce in a low carb flatbread, use in Chicken piccata, chicken alfredo, tacos, enchiladas, Indian Butter chicken, and more

Ground beef - Make a big burger and top with all sorts of things from cheese, to sauteed mushrooms, to grilled onions... or crumble and cook with taco seasoning and use in provolone cheese taco shells; throw in a dish with lettuce, avocado, cheese, sour cream for a tortilla-less taco salad

Almonds (plain or flavored) - these are a tasty and healthy snack; however, be sure to count them as you eat, because the carbs DO add up. Flavors include habanero, coconut, salt and vinegar and more.

The keto plan is a versatile and interesting way to lose weight, with lots of delicious food choices. Keep these 10 items stocked in your fridge, freezer, and larder, and you'll be ready to throw together some delicious keto meals and snacks at a moment's notice.

Weight Loss - Should You Indulge In Keto Snacks?

With so many people jumping onto the "ketogenic diet" bandwagon right now, more and more people are starting to wonder if this diet plan is for them. Even if you are not on a ketogenic diet, you would be hard pressed not to have seen keto specific food now popping up in your supermarket.

Marketers are onto the fact the ketogenic diet appears not to be going where they wanted it to and are starting to make "ready to go" keto friendly snacks. Should you indulge?

Here are some points to keep in mind about keto products:

1. Calories Matter. First, take note calories more than anything else matter here. Too many people dive into including keto snacks in their eating plan without so much as thinking about looking at the calorie count. If you eat a snack containing 400 calories that will need to be factored in somewhere!

Compare this to a non-traditional keto snack such as an apple at a 100 calories, and which do you think is better for your weight loss plan? You could even add some peanut butter to the apple to help better balance it out and you would still be under 200 calories, way less than the calories in the keto snack.

2. Keto Does Not Necessarily Mean "Weight Loss Friendly." Also, remember keto does not mean weight loss friendly. While many people use the ketogenic diet to lose weight, you still need to think about calories as just noted. Some people use this diet for health reasons, and many of these snacks are better marketed to them because they are not watching their calories so heavily.

Just because a product states it is keto does not necessarily mean it is designed to help you lose weight. The ketogenic diet is a low-carb, high-fat diet so it greatly lowers your carbohydrate intake, replacing it with fat.

3. Check The Nutrition. Finally, also keep nutrition in mind. If the keto snack is heavily processed as many are, and as one aims to replace some of the processed high carb snacks in their eating plan, they are still not always healthy. A chocolate bar is never a good choice, no matter if it is a keto bar or not. So do not lose common sense just because you see the term "keto."

If you keep these points in mind, you should be better prepared to decipher the marketing of keto products and ensure they do not steer you away from your smart course of eating healthily.

Although managing your disease can be very challenging, Type 2 diabetes is not a condition you must just live with. You can make simple changes to your daily routine and lower both your weight and your blood sugar levels. Hang in there, the longer you do it, the easier it gets.

How Long Does It Take to Get into Ketosis?

It takes a few days to a week on a keto diet before most people get into ketosis. This is because our bodies store a series of "emergency" carbohydrates in case we suddenly run out of bread and pasta.

If it's your first time getting into ketosis, you may not be sure what to expect. Some people have symptoms that suggest ketosis, while others don't notice any changes. The most common signs of ketosis for newbies are headache, fatigue and muscle cramps (symptoms of keto flu). Although unpleasant, this is a sign that you are reaching your goal.

So how do you know you're in ketosis if you don't have any symptoms? A common way to find out if you are in ketosis is to use a urine test for ketosis: it is the same concept that women use to perform a urine test to check if they are pregnant, but instead they will find out if you have managed to get into ketosis. .

When you are in ketosis, your urine will have a certain level of ketones (the fatty acid products that are broken down) that high carbohydrate diets do not get. This lets you know that you have achieved your goal. These urine bars are available online or at quality food stores.

You can also take a blood test to measure the same.

Knowing if you are in ketosis helps you understand if what you are eating is correct and will give you the certainty that you are doing things correctly. It is a great feeling to know that you are on your way to losing weight, becoming healthier and getting all the other benefits of the keto diet.

The good news is that you can start checking if ketosis occurs in your body only three days after starting the diet. Ketosis tests can be performed with the help of some products.

How to get into ketosis quickly

Ketosis is a natural state of the metabolic process. When a person has reached ketosis, his body burns stored fat instead of glucose.

As the body breaks down fat, acids called ketones begin to build up in the blood. These ketones then leave the body in the urine. The presence of ketones in the blood and urine indicates that a person has entered ketosis.

Ketosis can help a person lose unwanted fat, as the body begins to break down its fat stores instead of relying on carbohydrates for energy. In addition, some research suggests that ketosis can help suppress a person's appetite, which can also promote weight loss.

Achieving a state of ketosis isn't always easy. Many people who want to achieve ketosis stick to the keto diet. In this article, we discuss seven ways to quickly get into ketosis. We also examine the possible risks of putting the body in this metabolic state.

Top 3 tips for getting into ketosis quickly

Ways to bring the body into ketosis include:

1. Increased physical activity: a person can enter ketosis by increasing physical activity.

The more energy a person uses during the day, the more food he needs to eat for fuel.

Exercise helps a person to deplete the glycogen stores in his body. In most cases, glycogen stores are replenished when a person eats carbohydrates. If a person follows a low carbohydrate diet, he will not replenish his glycogen stores.

The body can take some time to learn how to use fat deposits instead of glycogen. A person can experience fatigue while his body regulates himself.

2. Significant reduction in carbohydrate intake: ketosis occurs when a lack of carbohydrates forces the body to use fat as a primary energy source instead of sugar.

A person trying to achieve ketosis, lose weight, reduce the risk of heart disease or maintain and control blood sugar levels, should try to reduce their carbohydrate intake to 20 grams (g) per day or less.

However, this is not a predetermined number. Some people can eat more carbohydrates and still go into a state of ketosis, while others will have to eat less.

3. Fasting for short periods.

Fasting or lack of food can help a person reach a state of ketosis. Many people can get into ketosis between meals.

CHAPTER FOUR

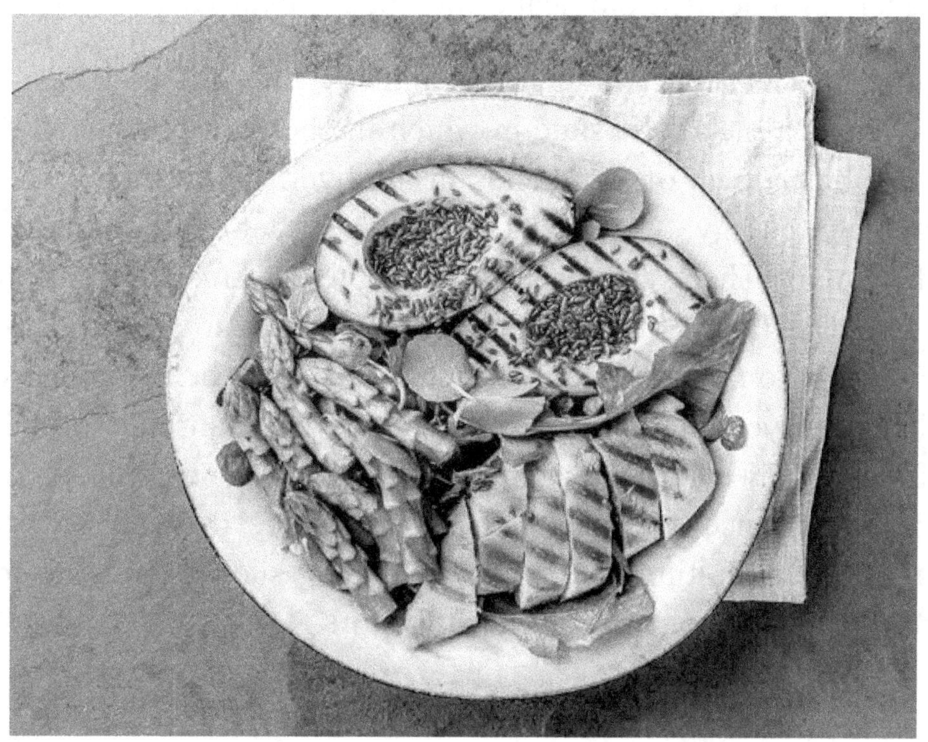

What are the effects of the ketogenic diet on behavior and cognition?

 Multiple forms of ketogenic diet (KD) have been used successfully for the treatment of drug-resistant epilepsy, however, its main use as first-line therapy is still limited. Additional research on its clinical efficacy and on the molecular basis of the activity will probably contribute to the reversal of any resistance to its implementation. In this review, we will try to clarify the current state of experimental and clinical data related to the neuroprotective and cognitive effects of coronary heart disease in humans and animals. In general, many research teams have shown that the effective implementation of KD has strong neuroprotective effects with respect to social behavior and cognition. We will also illustrate the role of KD in the interesting relationship between sleep, epilepsy and memory. Currently available evidence also indicates that, under proper supervision, and with additional studies studying long-term side effects, KD is also a relatively safe intervention, especially when compared to traditional antiepileptic drugs. In addition, due to its neuroprotective capacity, KD may also have a potential benefit for the treatment of other neurological or neurodegenerative disorders.

The ketogenic diet is a diet high in fat and low in carbohydrates that induces ketosis. Ketosis is a metabolic state in which the body uses ketone bodies, which consists of the breakdown of fatty acids in the liver, rather than carbohydrates as the main source of energy. Classic KD (cKD) has a fat / carbohydrate ratio plus a 3-4: 1 protein ratio. There are also less restrictive forms, such as the modified Atkins diet (MAD). In this diet, patients are encouraged to eat fat; However, there is no protein restriction. In addition, cKD and MAD can be integrated with long or medium chain triglycerides (LCT or MCT) to maintain the proper ratio and improve efficacy. The diets seem to be very effective since 36-85% of patients with epilepsy experience a seizure reduction of more than 50% when receiving treatment with KD. Multiple epileptic syndromes, such as glucose transporter 1 deficiency (GLUT1), are particularly sensitive to KD.

Cognitive effects of KD in epilepsy

Most KD studies focus on the impact of diet on seizure control. Less attention has been paid to the additional benefits of KD treatment, such as the effect on cognition. Parents of patients with epilepsy have reported cognitive improvement as one of the main motivators for starting and continuing KD disease. For example, Farasat and his colleagues showed that 90% of parents reported that cognitive improvement is a critical treatment goal. In addition, meeting the expectations of cognitive improvement was significantly correlated with a longer duration of the use of KD, while the objectives for seizure control and the reduction of non-anticonvulsant use. These findings highlight the importance of understanding the effects of KD on cognition in patients with epilepsy. The first randomized controlled controlled trial (RCT) that examined the behavioral and cognitive impact of KD disease in patients with epilepsy was recently published. However, there is no systematic overview of all clinical studies on the effects of KD disease on cognition in patients with epilepsy.

Although no prospective studies of evolutionary or behavioral outcomes have been performed so far, anecdotal evidence and measures of parental relationships have indicated that children treated with KD show greater alertness and better cognitive functioning, as well as better behavior. In addition to the diet regime itself and with special attention to pediatric cases, it has been shown that there is a significant therapeutic synergy between social behavioral support and Newcastle disease itself, suggesting that the involvement of emotional neurological pathways may Be a crucial factor in the efficacy of the disease.

What is the difference between healthy ketogenic diets and low carb diets?

One of the most common misconceptions is that a low carb diet is equivalent to a ketogenic diet. Both a low carb diet and a keto diet focus on eliminating carbohydrates, but there are some important differences between keto and low carb contcnt, as well as how they affect overall health. There is a good chance of meeting someone who swears bread with the same rigor that vegetarians avoid steak. It seems that low carb diets are the only way that people lose weight these days, and the high fat ketogenic plan is the most popular carbohydrate cutting method.

It is known that both keto and low carb diets offer rapid weight loss. But what is the difference between the two? While the keto diet is a low carb diet, it will still put you in a state of ketosis. People who follow a ketogenic diet should go into ketosis, since this is the condition in which the body burns fat as fuel instead of carbohydrates. In a state of ketosis, you tend to feel less hungry. The foods included in the keto diet and weight loss also help maintain muscle mass. This with the condition that you follow the diets with the correct technique.

Ketogenic diet vs low carb diet: what is the difference?

One of the most important steps in a keto diet is to limit your carbohydrate intake to a minimum of 20 grams per day. In addition, you should also limit your protein intake, depending on the level of your physical activity. A low carb diet, on the other hand, also requires that you limit carbohydrates, but it involves more protein than the keto diet. If you follow a low carb diet, 20% will include carbohydrates, 40% will contain protein and 40% will be fat. In a low carb diet, the body does not enter the state of ketosis. This type of diet offers temporary and rapid weight loss.

Low carb and keto diets are excellent for losing weight.

 However, a keto diet can simplify weight loss by keeping you satiated with fewer calories. One of the side effects of ketosis is the suppression of hunger. Ketones control ghrelin and cholecystokinin, two of the body's main hunger hormones. A ketogenic diet can help promote lasting hunger suppression by facilitating weight loss. In one study, 17 obese men received a keto diet (4% carbohydrates) or a low carb diet (35% carbohydrates), with no calorie restrictions on any diet.

Healthy Keto snacks for weight loss and health

Diet and exercise have been a big trend over the past three decades, although they have focused on rapid weight loss from diet pills and shock diets in recent years. However, over the past decade, more and more people have begun to understand that weight loss starts with a balanced diet of healthy snacks that includes all food groups with a regiment of regular exercises. Fewer people are taking whole categories out of their diet and focusing on eating the right foods for fat loss. Eating healthy snacks can be one of the most rewarding ways to lose weight while being able to enjoy a variety of foods.

Fruits are nutrient-rich weight loss snacks

Fruits are one of the few foods that offer a range of vitamins and minerals, while at the same time tasting absolutely delicious. Fruit, however, should always be fresh or at least frozen. Canned foods are considered processed foods and can contain an excessive amount of preservatives, syrups, extra sugars and other ingredients that produce a high calorie content, the benefits of the fruit itself.

Good weight loss snacks contain a variety of protein-containing foods that are vital for nuts. There are plenty of nuts available at the local grocery store, such as peanuts, nuts, pinpricks, macadamia nuts, sunflower seeds and more. Nuts are perfect fat loss snacks that are very convenient.

With so many healthy weight loss snacks to choose from, you can enjoy a variety of foods without sacrificing one particular group over another. While some healthy weight loss snacks can simply be low in fat, such as yogurt and cheese, some foods can benefit directly from other foods as well as antioxidants in teas. By creating a balanced meal plan with healthy weight loss snacks, people can enjoy a healthy lifestyle that contributes to a longer life.

How does Keto increase resistance?

At this point, you might think: "Friend, this matter of keto is too good to be true". It seems true, but believe me, once you're inside, you'll find all this 100% true.

Another great feature of the ketogenic diet is that it can significantly increase physical resistance. Your fat stores energy and keto and gives you constant access to all this energy.

The other way in which the body provides energy comes from stored carbohydrates. This is fortunate enough to do intensive exercise for a few hours. The stored fat is much better. Fat stores so much energy that it can stay for weeks or even months.

Most people are particularly good at burning carbohydrates. If this is the case, you can not reach your fat deposits, so they can not nourish your brain. What produces this? You must eat constantly before and immediately after long training sessions. Some people should also eat during training sessions. They also have to eat several times a day, just to keep them from getting angry. You know what the hacienda is. If you do not, it's when you're hungry + angry. It is a deadly combination and should be avoided at all costs. You may be familiar with when your partner is "angry."

So, if you're in ketosis, whether you're looking for mental focus or looking for a world-class athlete, ketosis gives you what you need to go where you want to be.

This is a dietary approach that works for many people, and here are 5 other benefits of ketogenic diets that you may not know about.

1 - Having kankose means that the body can process fat and use it as fuel in a way that no other state allows. Carbohydrates are much easier to convert and use as fuel, so if you give a lot to your body, you should burn them and use them before your body begins to develop and use the fat as fuel.

2 - Another advantage of being in a state of ketosis is that excess ketones are not harmful to your system. All the key tones that you create and that your body does not need are excreted simply and safely in the urine. In fact, this excellent benefit is the reason why you can check if you are in a state of ketosis in the morning by using urine test strips.

3 - When your body gets used to being in ketosis, it actually starts giving preference to ketones for glucose. This is the ideal state in which you want your body to be: it no longer needs sugar, and in fact it prefers protein as a source of fuel instead of sugar.

4 - Another advantage of weight loss through the ketogenic diet is that being in a ketogenic state is very useful for regulating insulin levels in the body. Insulin is one of the substances that makes you want food, especially because it is rich in sugar. This is why insulin is one of the most important elements of weight loss and is good for your health.

5 - Last but not least, most people who use a ketogenic diet say they are in a ketogenic state and feel much less hungry than when they are in a non-ketogenic state. It is much easier to follow a diet, a diet, if you do not fight against hunger and cravings at every step. In fact, feeling hungry can often be what derails someone's best efforts. If you are not involved, it is easier to achieve your goals in general.

Now that you are aware of all the benefits of losing weight in a state of ketosis, it is logical that you try this approach after all, what do you have to lose except weight?

Ketogenic diet necessary for children?

The ketogenic diet actually started as a treatment for children with epilepsy. This dietary method rich in fats and carbohydrates is used in medicine to help control the activity of seizures. The typical model provides 3-4 grams of fat per 1 gram of carbohydrates and proteins. This strategy is often used when a child has not responded to anticonvulsant drugs. It is carefully planned and monitored by a medical team. Following its medical origins, the keto diet became a conventional method of losing weight. By following a ketogenic diet, your body goes into a metabolic state called ketosis. Instead of burning carbohydrates for fuel, your body starts burning its own fat. To achieve this, carbohydrate intake must be extremely low, typically less than 20-30 grams of carbohydrates per day. An apple is equivalent to about 20 grams of carbohydrates. For this reason, fruit is not allowed in the keto diet.

How long do children need a ketogenic diet for?

You should know if a ketogenic diet works for your child within a few months. If so, the doctor may recommend stopping the baby's diet after 2 years of seizure control. The weaning process is carried out for several months to avoid the activation of seizures.

Ketosis treatment process for children:

Hospital treatment with the keto diet for children with epilepsy may begin with a controlled medical fast for one or two days. Fasting helps speed up the creation of ketones. Other programs can avoid fasting and instead gradually increase fat intake for a few days. Medical staff will monitor closely during this period to make sure there are no adverse changes. After this phase, the child may be given keto shakes to drink before switching to solid foods. A medical team that includes a registered dietitian, doctor and registered nurse usually participates to prevent the child from having nutritional deficiencies and having no negative side effects. The team will also instruct parents on how to integrate the diet into the child's daily life and how to check urine for ketones and how to check if there are other products in the home that may contain carbohydrates, such as mouthwashes, toothpaste and medications. . These small things are important when following a ketogenic diet for medical reasons. This process can take about 1-2 weeks. If the diet is successful and the child's parents can monitor and help them follow the diet well enough at home, the children can take fewer medications for their condition. Regular checks are carried out to check metabolism and seizure control.

Children should be offered nutrient-dense foods with carbohydrates, including vegetables, fruits, whole grains, legumes, beans and dairy products such as milk to meet their carbohydrate needs. Carbohydrate foods that have a lower nutritional value and should be minimally included include foods with added sugar, sugary drinks and foods with highly processed or refined carbohydrates.

"The best dietary guide advises children to follow a diversified diet that provides them with the right amount of all the nutrients, macro and micro, that their growing bodies need. This includes a wide range of fruit, vegetables, cereals, half of which must be whole grains and dairy products. Many of these are prohibited or severely restricted in the ketogenic diet.

CHAPTER FIVE

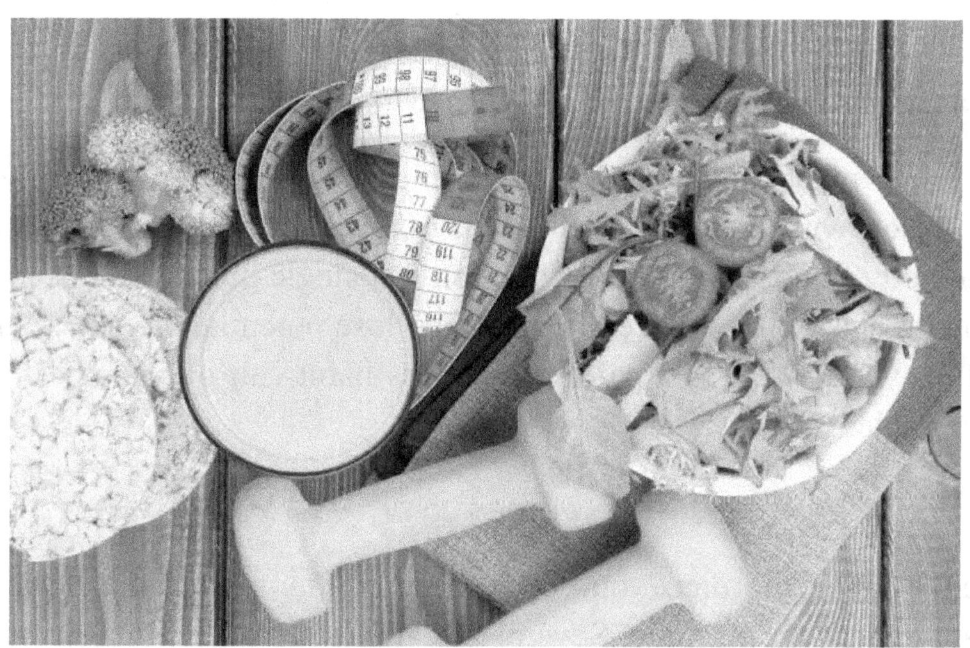

Effective Keto weight loss plan

Getting fit and healthy is very important for getting the desired weight loss without sacrificing your daily lifestyle and health. In this article I will educate you on three habits for effective weight loss.

1. Eat healthy

Eating a healthy diet for life will not only give you a healthier body, but a more faithful body as well. Eating more vegetables, fruits and other high-fibre foods are crucial to your weight loss plan, as these foods can burn fat easily. The fibre content fills your stomach tight, making you feel fuller and fuller, thus avoiding unwanted snacks. Nutrients and vitamins, you get from vegetables and fruits will also prevent you from developing feared diseases such as heart disease and cancer.

2. Regular exercise

The regular exercise program is not new to us, but the problem is discipline. If you're not mentally ready to do a regular fitness activity, you definitely won't miss those extra bumps on your belly. Exercise comes in many forms and that's what makes this habit fun. All physical activities such as dancing, sports, swimming, walking, jogging, biking or even normal morning car wash can contribute to your workout routine.

3. A daily dose of meditation

Meditation is a practice that helps relax the mind and body with powerful techniques. Once you focus on meditation, you also apply a good posture that forms a fine body figure. Actually, meditation is a single practice that can not only give you health and wellness potential, but also lose potential weight. Maintaining a healthy lifestyle as well as a safe weight loss habit can overcome all kinds of weight loss problems.

How to implement keto diet

When using a ketogenic diet, your body becomes more of a fat-burner than a carbohydrate-dependent machine. Several researches have linked the consumption of increased amounts of carbohydrates to development of several disorders such as diabetes and insulin resistance. By nature, carbohydrates are easily absorbable and therefore can be also be easily stored by the body. Digestion of carbohydrates starts right from the moment you put them into your mouth. As soon as you begin chewing them, amylase (the enzymes that digest carbohydrate) in your saliva is already at work acting on the carbohydrate-containing food.

In the stomach, carbohydrates are further broken down. When they get into the small intestines, they are then absorbed into the bloodstream. On getting to the bloodstream, carbohydrates generally increase the blood sugar level. This increase in blood sugar level stimulates the immediate release of insulin into the bloodstream. The higher the increase in blood sugar levels, the more the amount of insulin that is release. Insulin is a hormone that causes excess sugar in the bloodstream to be removed in order to lower the blood sugar level. Insulin takes the sugar and carbohydrate that you eat and stores them either as glycogen in muscle tissues or as fat in adipose tissue for future use as energy.

However, the body can develop what is known as insulin resistance when it is continuously exposed to such high amounts of glucose in the bloodstream. This scenario can easily cause obesity as the body tends to quickly store any excess amount of glucose. Health conditions such as diabetes and cardiovascular disease can also result from this condition. Keto diets are low in carbohydrate and high in fat and have been associated with reducing and improving several health conditions.

Test for Ketosis

I often have people email me wanting to know how they can tell if they've reached ketosis or not. Because one of the goals of medifast is to consume a low enough amount of carbs and calories and a high enough amount of protein to get your body burning fat rather than carbs. Most people want to get to this state as soon as possible because this is when you begin to see the results. So how can you tell if you've reached these levels? Well, you can look at your physical symptoms, you can test yourself, or you can do both. I will discuss this more in the following article.

The first thing that you might notice is that you're having an easier time on the diet. The cravings might become less and you might find that you're just not as hungry. You might also find that you have a bit more energy. I've also heard people say that they noticed a change in their breath. They've said that their breath had an almost fruity, sweet smell and / or taste.

Using Strips To Test If You Are In Ketosis Or Not: If you doubt these symptoms or just want to be sure that you've finally reached this state, you can use little strips that test for ketones in your urine. These are often sold under names like ketostix or ketone strips. Basically, you urinate onto the end of the stick and then wait for the amount of time indicated in the directions. (This is usually anywhere from 15 - 30 seconds. It does not take long to get results.) Usually you are looking for the strips to turn color. The strips come with directions that will show you what color you are looking for. But with many, you are wanting the strip to turn a purple to dark pink color to indicate that you are in ketosis.You can get the strips at most pharmacies and grocery stores. They are often in the diabetic section. You don't need a prescription for them, but they are sometimes kept behind the counter, depending on the store.

What happens if you don't see the change in color? Well, there are a few possibilities. The first would be that you're not yet showing ketones in your urine. You can try to check again in a few days. Sometimes, if you work out heavily, your muscles will need the ketones as fuel and therefore it won't be in your urine. You may also have been drinking so much water that your urine is too diluted to change the color.

I understand that ketosis is really where you want to be on medifast and I know that we all want validation that we are there. But the strips really are a guide. If you are seeing some of the symptoms and the weight is coming off as it should, there really is not reason to give so much importance to the test results or to let them stress you out. What is really important is getting the results on the scale, not in the strips, although they can help to offer you some reassurance if you need it.

How to lose weight on keto diet

When you start eating more fats and eliminating all the extra carbohydrates (sugar, bread and pasta), you tend to stop feeling the fluctuations in blood sugar that plague most people on the standard American diet. When your body uses ketones as fuel, it has a constant supply of energy in the form of body fat. When your body depends on glucose, you need a regular intake of carbohydrates to maintain it.

Ketones can control their hunger and satiety hormones so that they are full and full. This means less cravings, more energy and an increase in fat burning. Is that how it works.

Effective weight loss is more than just a food

Make sure you get enough sleep

Researchers note that you can compromise your weight loss efforts if you don't get enough sleep every night. The main problem with too little sleep is that your metabolism is trying to compensate for the lack of energy by slowing down, which means that your body will convert the food you eat into energy at a slower pace. Small group studies have shown that people who sleep less than necessary are more likely to eat more and convert fewer calories into energy when doing the same activities. Therefore, for effective weight loss, you need to get enough sleep.

Eat more varied foods

Another secret to losing weight efficiently is eating more varied foods. If you eat the same food every day and every meal, not only will you be bored with it, but you will also be tempted to eat more to make up for the hunger you will feel. It seems that both humans and animals tend to eat less, in quantity, if they are offered greater diversity of food to eat. So instead of loading your plate with just one type of food, add more foods to the same plate, and you will see how easy it will be to lose weight while eating less.

Effective weight loss is about attitude

It is very important to have the right mindset when starting a diet or to promise to live healthier and lose weight. If you drop what you think about food and remove it from the equation, don't be surprised when you notice that things don't work that way. What you need is a positive attitude; you will have to change the way you think about food and focus on healthy options. Over time, your mentality will become an ally in the fight against extra pounds, and it will be much easier for you to lose weight.

The best calorie-free drink: water

Drinking water is important when you want to lose weight. A great quality of natural water is that it helps the body eliminate toxins and especially sodium, which is the main culprit when you feel bloated for no apparent reason. Carbonated drinks should be out of the question when considering effective weight loss, but water should always be abundant and readily available.

Worry less

Last but not least, effective weight loss strategies should also include less stress. When he is stressed, he tends to eat more than usual to compensate for what he feels. Instead of feeding blues with unhealthy foods, consider starting over with the right foods with a healthier lifestyle.

When it comes to losing weight, there aren't two people alike, it's about what works for you, but if you put the tips in this article into practice, you will get remarkable results.

Staying Motivated for Weight Loss: Three Fundamental Diet Rules for Effective Weight Loss

There is no question about this. The promise of a new diet is very exciting and powerful. Expectations for success are high. But despite that initial burst of energy and enthusiasm, why does our motivation to lose weight disappear, and we only go back to old habits weeks later?

Regardless of past experience, there is good news. You can find a new way of eating that will not bore you. If you first understand that typical "diets" as we know them don't work and that your efforts to lose fat must involve a lifestyle change, then you've discovered a key secret to truly effective weight loss. You just have to know what to look for when considering a new diet plan, and your continued weight loss success is yours.

Tip 1: be satisfied

The common belief among dieters is that hunger is a key strategy to lose pounds. This belief could not be more wrong, so the vast majority of diets end up failing. Remember, the best diet is a lifestyle change in the way you eat. Being hungry all the time is not something you can keep for a lifetime. When your stomach growls and is weak with hunger, those old habits will eventually creep back.

Your level of hunger must be manageable. That is why experts recommend eating between 1,300 and 2,000 calories per day to lose weight, with a preference for the high end. By the way, they also agree that it is easier to be more active than to skip food to achieve the same calorie reduction. Keep calories at a sustainable level and move more, and you won't have to starve.

If you're eating a reasonable amount but still hungry, try adding more protein, fiber, and healthy fats to your diet. You'll feel fuller longer, and your body will appreciate the extra nutrition.

Tip 2: make room for the foods you like

Yes, your eating habits require a change in lifestyle, but straying too far from your normal diet can be a major blow to your motivation for weight loss and ultimate success. For example, if you love meat, following a vegetarian diet is probably not enough. And those who love whole grains and fruits probably won't be too excited about a low-carb diet (which is a fundamentally bad diet to start with). Fortunately, there is no need to sacrifice. Healthy and effective weight loss has room for all kinds of taste preferences.

Tip 3: welcome variety

Does eating low-calorie diet shakes and bars seem like something you can do, let alone want to do, for the rest of your life? Our brains and bodies crave variety, and since it's that very important spice of life, adding different foods to your lifestyle plan keeps the flames of motivation to lose weight and maintain a healthy weight. That burns quickly. In addition to boredom, our bodies need food from many different sources for optimal health. There are many whole foods to explore. Don't deny yourself!

There are other reasons why choosing a lifestyle carefully is better than staying motivated to lose weight. However, these three tips should help lay the foundation for any effective weight loss effort. Satisfaction, fun, and variety. Don't you think it is a better way to live a happy and healthy life?

CHAPTER SIX

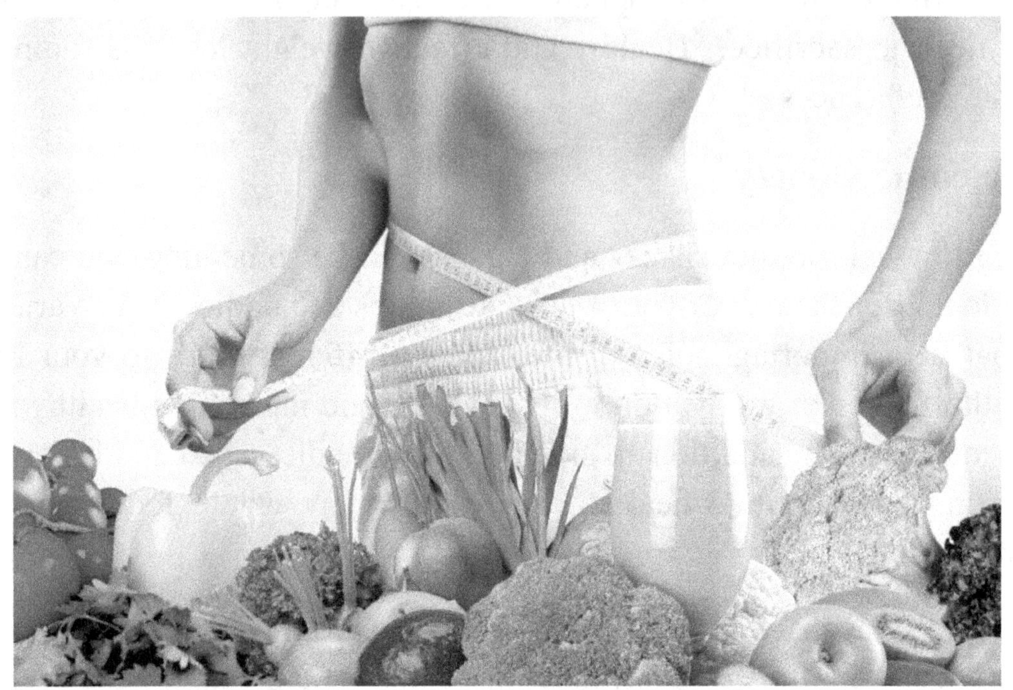

General effective weight loss plan

With the convenience of technology, obesity has quickly become the problem of most people in modern days. Especially with automation structures such as elevators, escalators, and efficient transport systems, people drastically reduce their chances of exercise. In addition to this problem, the modern diet rich in fats and carbohydrates has worsened the problem considerably. Maintaining an ideal weight has become a challenge. Hence, a total approach to weight loss is essential to combat the problem of obesity. It is the ultimate solution for sustainable weight control instead of a diet that slows down your metabolism. Once you stop staying, your weight will skyrocket quickly. In a yo-yo syndrome, it is more harmful.

So how to plan and execute an effective weight loss plan?

Mentality and determination

You have to stick to a strong reason why you need to lose that weight. The extra reasons you can think of in the end will give you more support. As motivation gets stronger, execution will become easier later. Next, you need to determine the ideal weight you want to reach. Use a visual form as an indicator, e.g., like a particular size of dress or shirt that you want to wear eventually. Imagine adapting to that outfit and experiencing excitement and happiness. When you manage to associate a strong emotion of the image with achieving your goal, you will have a stronger inspiration to follow with your plan during the execution.

Keep a diary

Record all the food you eat and the time you eat it in a notebook. It also records the amount of time you spend doing exercise and sitting idle (for example, sitting in front of the TV). By scoring, you strengthen your determination towards your goal. It will also help you adjust and revise your plan later. The more detail it is, the more effective it will be.

Plan a gradual weight loss plan

It will make your trip more pleasant. This is very critical since it avoids the possibility of yo-yo syndrome. Another important reason for doing this is due to medical reasons. It is always dangerous to lose weight drastically, as your metabolic system will be completely altered. You may no get have enough food nutrition for your body to function properly. Losing weight very fast is not a good thing. With much more gradual planning, it will also give you the necessary encouragement along the way, as the goal is much easier to achieve and less likely to give up. You can always improve your plan later when your body can easily make changes.

Plan your diet

This is the most important aspect of an effective weight loss plan. You will probably train one to three times a week. However, you will take at least twenty meals (based on a three meal per day diet). Since the diet is a very complex segment, we will discuss it in detail along the way.

Plan your exercise

An exercise is an important approach to weight loss. Always set a gradual goal. You have to condition your heart slowly. In fact, a lower intensity, but prolonged for a longer duration, will eventually burn more fat. It also gives you better motivation, as it is more feasible. Also, when you train to train more often, you also find it easier to get into the habit of exercising. Always start with a simple form of exercise, like cycling. It is also more convenient to perform an exercise where you can train on a cycling machine while watching TV.

Check your result every two weeks and improve your plan

Since most weight loss takes time, don't be anxious to monitor your results on a daily basis, as it will demoralize you. If you can, reward yourself on the way. It will keep you motivated and stick to your plan.

There are no shortcuts to sustainable weight loss in a healthy way. A slow and steady way will entertain you in losing weight and, therefore, will give you a lot of motivation to carry out your plan. A master plan is needed to ensure long-term success.

Discover Liquid Diet As An Extraordinary Effective Weight Loss Secret

The liquid diet is an incredible secret to effective weight loss that has been shown to be very helpful for quick and significant results. They are now used very frequently by those who want to lose excess weight quickly. They simply include meal plans that exclude solid foods but only incorporate liquids like; water, herbal teas, fruit juices, vegetable juices, and other nutritional shakes.

However, aside from its important benefits in quick and easy weight loss, here are five healthier benefits of this type of diet.

1. Help flush toxins out of the body: Toxins are dangerous and unwanted waste materials found in the body. They become harmful if not removed regularly, and liquid diets like vegetable/water juices help flush toxins out of the body.

2. Helps rejuvenate skin: When you embark on liquid diets, it makes your skin younger and healthier. This change in appearance can be evident in just 24 hours after starting the diet. This is one of the reasons why liquid diets are endorsed by most celebrities and have gained so much popularity.

3. It helps digestion: we all know that liquids are digested faster than solid foods. In the case of liquid diets, since liquids are easier to digest than solids, the digestive system is not overloaded as digestion occurs.

4. The liquid diet improves your memory. They act as memory boosters, especially with diets containing herbal teas, vegetable juices, and fruit juices that contain so many useful nutrients/vitamins.

5. Increase your energy levels: You will notice a noticeable increase in vitality and energy when you embark on liquid diets. This is largely due to the nutritional value of the dietary elements.

These benefits demonstrate that liquid slimming diets are essential for you, especially if you want to get very fast results. This really is an extraordinary secret to effective weight loss.

Do not exercise during this particular type of diet. You should only participate in relaxing walks as a form of exercise.

Liquid diets are very effective. However, you should only do this for a short period of time due to the fact that the diet strictly limits certain calories, and this may not be good for your health if maintained for a long period of time.

It is advisable to use a suitable diet plan for better guidance on how to use this secret to lose weight effectively.

Nutritional tips for effective weight loss

Simply following a diet will present temporary weight loss. However, for effective weight loss, you must learn to follow a lifelong eating plan. You should aim to eat quality food and increase the amount of energy you burn.

Quality foods are foods that have more thick fiber and fodder to make you feel full faster, foods with lower levels of fat and sugar, and foods that are not refined or processed.

Be sure to eat small but frequent meals throughout the day, where all meals should have some protein to help maintain your muscles and energy levels. Also, eat more fruits and vegetables daily for your daily vitamin and mineral needs.

To find out how many calories it takes each day to lose weight, you must multiply your weight in pounds by twelve calories. If you are looking for weight maintenance, you must multiply your weight by 15 calories.

Once you know how many calories you need per day, you can work to reduce your daily calorie intake to lose weight. However, don't go below the required amount of calories for your body, so as not to go into starvation mode where your body lowers your metabolic rate and then starts to accumulate fat instead of burning it.

At the same time, you find an increase in hunger pangs where you begin to crave high-energy foods that you really should avoid. Rather, it tries to reduce consumption of foods with obvious and hidden fats, while avoiding severe dietary restrictions.

However, you should be aware of when you overeat, so that you can exercise later and burn off excess calories as compensation. Instead of managing your weight, start managing your body fat levels with the goal of moderate fat loss of one pound per week.

Benefits of stretching for effective weight loss

In order to work effectively during any physical activity such as exercise, the muscles must be stretched and extended. Stretching is a variety of exercises in which muscles are used to help condition a person's body to adapt to physical activities. Although some disagree that stretching is of some importance for improving health, other specialists believe that the benefits of stretching may offer progress in the development of weight loss.

Any form of exercise, such as stretching, offers many beneficial factors for a person's health. There are benefits of stretching for an effective weight loss process, which include; healthy blood distribution, burning additional calories, toned muscles, and more flexibility. Including stretching in regular training, the regimen can greatly improve the process and speed up results.

Healthy distribution of blood

Healthy blood distribution develops during a stretching activity. The pumping action of the muscles causes the blood to pass through the veins and into the heart, increasing the amount of oxygen that is distributed to the muscles. This process helps improve a person's ability to perform any physical activity such as exercise.

Burn extra calories

Calories are burned during stretching, it may not be much in contrast to cardiovascular exercises, but it is better than not exercising at all. Calories burned during stretching can build up in the long run when more intense stretches are performed.

Toned muscles

Developing and toning the muscles of the body results in a faster metabolism. Many stretching exercises aim to build core, leg, and arm muscles. Building these muscles can help strengthen the body and also further increase the rate at which the body burns calories, resulting in faster weight loss.

Improve flexibility

Improving the body's ability to be flexible can improve a person's ability to perform effortlessly and use their body in many physical activities. Constant stretching can gradually extend the muscles to use them efficiently.

In general, without an adequate diet and an active lifestyle, weight loss cannot be achieved. By adding regular stretching exercises before, during, or after a training program, the weight loss process can be improved along with the wonderful benefits of stretching.

Understand body type and body shape to lose weight and stay fit

We often wonder why some people lose weight very quickly while struggling. Sometimes we also find it hard to understand how and why some people don't have to do anything for an exceptional physique, or always look elegant, regardless of what they wear. Well, it's time to discover for yourself and find out what you can do to make your body look perfect for you.

The truth behind our differences in the body was discovered by a psychologist, dr. William H Sheldon, during the 1940s. After years of study, he concluded that we all inherit one of the three basic types of the human body. He identified these body types as:

1) Endomorphic: This person has a chubby/stocky build. They build muscle and body fat easily but have a hard time losing weight.

2) Ectomorph: This person has a generally thin and delicate build. They do not get fat easily and also have difficulty gaining weight

3) Mesomorphic: This person has a robust/muscular build. Rapidly increase muscles and fats, but also lose weight easily

Biologically, women are more likely to have a curvy body shape due to levels of the female hormone (estrogen) in their bodies, which promote fat storage.

However, our body shapes still vary quite significantly. This is due to the food we eat and the physical activity in which we participate or not.

There are at least four common body shapes, and each has its own advantages and risk factors that need to be considered for weight loss and fitness, which are:

1) The apple: It has a bigger chest and belly with narrow hips and thighs. It is very likely that they are an endomorph or a mesomorph.

Apple-shaped men and women are typically rounded, but when muscular, they have a funnel-like (inverted triangle) appearance. Apples easily increase body fat, but for men, this is balanced by the high presence of testosterone, which aids metabolism.

Health studies have shown that apple-shaped men and women may be more prone to cardiovascular disease and metabolic disorders like diabetes. This is due to increased stress on the heart and digestive system.

Preferred fitness regimes for the apple body shape involve longer workouts for the chest and waist. Squats, push-ups, stair climbing, are an example of simple and effective exercises for Apple.

Other recommended exercises include tennis, team sports, running, biking, or swimming for at least 40 minutes, 3-4 times per week. We also recommend Pilates to tone your life.

2) The pear: It has a narrow chest and a waist with wider hips and bigger buttocks. They must be primarily a mesomorph. The pear has a vase shape, which in some cultures was associated with fertility. Pears tend to grow and lose weight easily, especially on the hips.

Regarding health, pears are said to be less prone to cardiovascular disease and diabetes, as most of the body fat is stored in the thighs and buttocks. This, however, is not a reason to avoid cardiovascular training.

The tendency of most pears is to aggressively train the thighs and buttocks to burn fat. This, in fact, only increases the size of the muscles, making the thighs and buttocks appear larger. Fitness experts recommend cardiovascular exercises, racket sports, leg lifts, low resistance cycling as great ways to tone and balance your upper and lower body.

3) The hourglass: It has a wide chest and wide hips with a narrow waist. They are likely to be endomorphic or even mesomorphic.

The hourglass has a voluptuous body shape, commonly considered the classic female. They gain weight easily, and some (not all) have a hard time losing it.

As more fat is stored in the upper (chest) and lower (hip) areas, hourglasses may be less prone to metabolic disturbances, while more prone to cardiovascular disease.

For fitness, cardiovascular endurance exercises (e.g., running, light resistance cycling, swimming, team sports) are recommended 3-4 times per week. Also, pilates and back exercises are great for maintaining an upright posture and a slim beltline.

4) The banana: it has a few variations between the size of the chest, the waist, and the hips. I am usually an ectomorph.

The shape of the banana is sometimes known as a ruler. This body shape easily loses weight and effort to build muscle.

Bananas do not fatten easily, but when they do, they tend mainly around the abdomen (waist) and buttocks. Excessive weight gain around the waist increases the risk of metabolic disorders.

The recommended fitness exercises are intended to promote muscle development. They include pilates, walking, jogging on steep climbs, push-ups, sit-ups, squats, and bench presses.

Effective weight loss with herbs

Although herbs have been used as traditional medicines for many years, modern societies are just beginning to realize the effectiveness of these herbs. In fact, losing weight can be difficult unless you know the best approach. Using natural herbs is a good place to start because effective weight loss with herbs ensures that you are losing weight in a way that is not harmful to your body. There are many herbs on the market; Consider some of these herbs known to help you achieve your weight loss goals.

Herbs to suppress appetite

Guarana acts as a stimulant for the nervous system. This herb contains guaranine, which helps relax the body, reduces the feeling of depression, and increases the resistance of the body. Thanks to its properties, guarana is effective in suppressing emotional nutrition triggered by sensations of stress. If left unchecked, emotional consumption can significantly affect your weight loss goals.

Guar gum comes from guar beans. Guar gum has the ability to suppress appetite, increase metabolism rate, restore good cholesterol, and stabilize blood sugar levels. What makes guar gum an effective herb for weight loss is that it slows down the digestive process and gives you the feeling of being full for a longer period.

Flaxseed is effective for losing weight naturally. Flaxseed is full of essential fats that the body requires to perform its physiological functions. This means that when consuming flax seeds, the body does not crave fatty foods, which are primarily responsible for unhealthy weight gain. The reason your body craves fatty foods is that it lacks the essential nutrient fats provided by herbs such as flax seeds.

Metabolic Herbs

Green tea contains compounds that improve your body's metabolism rate so that the body can convert fats into energy at a much faster rate. Incorporate green tea into your diet regularly to experience its weight loss benefits. Stubborn weight gain is often due to the body's low metabolism. This means that your body digests food too quickly and burns fat too slowly, causing an excessive build-up of unwanted fat.

Natural spices like cayenne pepper, bell pepper, spicy mustard, turmeric, and chili pepper help regulate the body's metabolism. Spices warm the body, increase blood circulation, and speed up the rate at which fats break down into energy. Use these species daily by spraying your healthy diet.

Regulatory Herbs

Ginger root encourages the digestive system to produce enzymes that aid the proper digestion of food. The production of these enzymes means that the food you eat completely breaks down (increased metabolism) and is absorbed uniformly in the body.

Ginseng is a natural root that helps relieve chronic fatigue. The herb is used to restore the body's endurance and increase its energy after a period of emotional or physical stress. Ginseng also provides you with the energy to train regularly and have a healthier existence.

 Numerous weight loss programs exist, all claiming their effectiveness. But a good number of these weight loss programs, supplements, and diets are diets that can be harmful to health. It is true that effective herbal weight loss does not happen overnight, but you will start to see better results that will last longer. Keep in mind that even the best herbs won't work as well if you don't commit to regular exercise and a healthy diet.

CHAPTER SEVEN

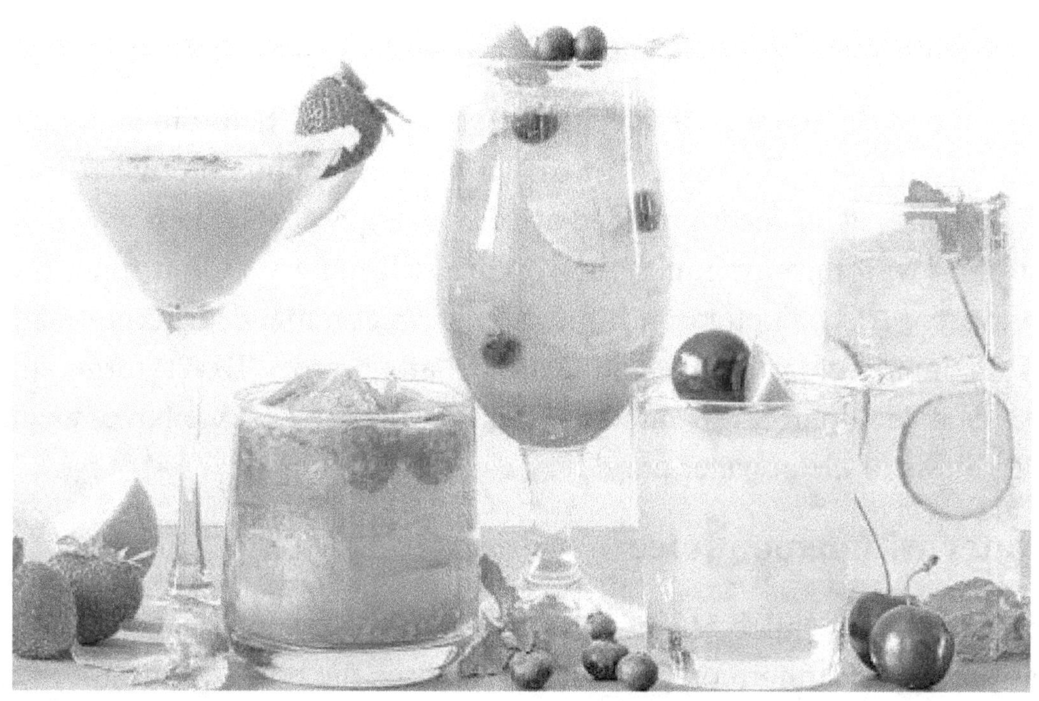

The effective keto approved drinks to lose weight

We all know that the way to lose weight and gain a good body is mainly through proper nutrition and regular exercise. You should pay attention not only to what you eat but also to what you drink. After all, 80% of our water (liquid) and 20% of our daily calories enter our bodies through the unhealthy drinks in which we participate. Sometimes this 20% would be enough to start gaining weight. So in this article, I will tell you what drinks to drink to lose weight or just to keep you in great shape.

Some drinks can help you lose weight and keep your body in shape. It will calm your appetite and cleanse your body with these helpful weight loss drinks. And above all, they are all-natural and easy to prepare at home without spending a lot of money. The most effective weight loss drinks

1. water

If you decide to lose weight and keep your body toned, reconsider your attitude towards water. Water is a panacea for weight loss without side effects. The water is free and contains no calories. It attenuates the appetite and energizes the body.

In fact, hunger and thirst are generated in the same part of the brain and are caused by the same histamine. This makes it difficult to distinguish between thirst and hunger. Therefore, it is recommended to drink a glass of water when you are hungry and then wait thirty minutes. If you are still hungry at that time, then you are very hungry. Also, doctors and nutritionists recommend drinking a glass of water half an hour before meals and 2 hours afterward. Don't forget that the human body is made up of 80% water and that to look the best we have, we need to drink 1.5-2.5 liters of clean water per day.

2. Hot water with lemon juice

Hot water with lemon juice is an excellent slimming drink that speeds up the weight loss process. Furthermore, this drink cleanses the body, ridding it of toxins. Lemon is an excellent health stimulant and can harmonize the body. It is no secret that lemon contains vitamins A, B2, C, pectin, carotene, and various trace elements. Lemon helps us reduce blood sugar levels and stimulates our liver to burn fat.

3. Green tea

Green tea has been famous for its medicinal properties. Green tea helps preserve youth and slimness. After drinking a cup of green tea, you will feel an increase in energy and a suppression of appetite. This is the only drink that burns calories immediately and does so at a rate of 70-90 kcal per cup.

4. Herbal teas

Everyone knows that there are many herbs with medicinal qualities. Herbs not only help improve health, but they can also eliminate excess weight. The simplest and most effective weight loss teas are peppermint and chamomile. Both teas relieve appetite, tone the body, help with proper digestion and metabolism, and help eliminate the stress that can occur due to excess weight.

5. Ginger tea

Ginger tea is one of the best drinks for weight loss and has great benefits for the body. It is no wonder that ginger is called universal medicine. This root is one of the most valuable spices in the world, and ginger tea helps to remove excess weight from the body. Ginger tea accelerates metabolism, strengthens the immune system, tones, tones, and cleanses the body.

6. Fresh fruit juices

Freshly squeezed healthy fruit and vegetable juices are not only tasty and healthy, but they also have plenty of vitamins and help in the battle to lose weight. The most effective slimming juices are grapefruit, orange, mandarin, apple, blueberry, and tomato. All these juices will help you burn fat.

How to structure an effective weight loss training routine

Instead of shooting for a great weight loss exercise routine, a well-toned and healthy physique, people are obsessed with shifting numbers on the scale, which is the wrong strategy.

Your overall appearance and well-being are determined by numerous factors; These are also responsible for independently guiding an individual's total weight.

You can be "light" but be free and flabby, 100% out of shape and in bad health; Likewise, it is possible to be "heavy" but thin, thin and in exceptional health. There are very "light" people who are in terrible health with a smooth, loose and flabby physique, as well as out of shape.

The reading on the scale is actually a sum of the load driven by fat, muscle, water, and glycogen. Choosing a simple "weight loss" tactic is, in effect, flying blindly, because it does not take into account each of these factors, which are the ratio of an individual's total weight.

In order to lose "bad" weight and maintain "good" weight, you need to undertake an efficient weight-loss exercise routine, which will help you achieve your primary goal of achieving lean by cutting back with an energetic physique. The main goal of the weight loss exercise routine should be.

Reduce body fat and preserve lean muscle mass. This is truly the only way to have a well-formed physique and good long-term results. Drop that figure on the scale! Instead, devote your time and effort to a high-quality weight loss exercise routine that works to reduce unwanted fat and also maintain lean mass.

The amount of lean and healthy muscles you have decides your basal metabolic rate or the number of calories a person burns while resting. The higher the muscle tissue, the higher the metabolism rate, and the greater the amount of excess fat burned.

Many of you want to have a slim, firm, and well-toned body; The muscle you develop will allow you to achieve that same aspiration. A reduction in body fat percentage without adequate muscle mass growth will be negligible to help an individual achieve a torn and toned body.

You have to recognize that "fast diets" can help you lose weight quickly, even if the results don't last long and, therefore, will surely fail. These extreme diets will force the body to break down lean mass, thereby reducing metabolism.

Your "lighter" body will certainly lack muscle tone along with strength. Plus, it was programmed to store fat, calling it almost certain that you can expect to return to the original weight, if not more.

In a "weight loss" approach that helps reduce excess fat while preserving the muscles. A highly effective weight loss exercise routine will guarantee it. A good weight loss exercise routine is actually a well-formulated way to restructure your body, lose fat, maintain it, and get a toned and athletic body.

Exceed your weight number as it would reflect on the scale; alternatively, focus on your weight loss training routine, which has major consequences.

How to eat to lose weight effectively

Everyone seems to be trying to lose weight at one point or another in their lives, some more than others. There are a million different diets and exercise plans that promise to make you lose five inches, drop two sizes of clothing, or burn two thousand calories a day. But the fact is, regardless of what you choose to do regarding a diet or plan, you still have to eat. Food is necessary for survival, simple and clear. The fact is, you must eat smart and make the right decisions in order to achieve effective weight loss and achieve your body's goals. In addition to what you put in your body, how and when you eat is the most important thing. Here are some tips to help you make your decisions to help you lose more weight.

Five small meals

Smaller meals more often are really better for you because you will eat less and therefore be less tempted to swallow unnecessary calories, and your body will be able to process food more efficiently. Five small food instead of two or three large meals allow you to eat more things that you love, too, because you can control your portions more easily since hunger will not be your main thought.

Eat on side-sized plates or lunch

The size of your plate can affect the amount of food you eat. Firstly, it can't fit as much on a smaller plate, so portions will have to be smaller. Therefore, the psychological aspect will prevent you from coming back for a few seconds because this would mean that you have eaten too much as you are trying to lose weight, and a second help would be contradictory to your goal.

Take your time

It takes at least fifteen minutes for the brain to process the food it is eating and tell it that the stomach is full. Therefore, if you eat fast, you could never understand that you are eating too much because your brain will not be able to tell you in time. But if you take the time to chew each bite and breathe for a minute or two, you can tell where your body is and if it really wants more food.

Drink the water first

Drink ice-cold water before eating. Coldwater will force your body to start digesting it, as you will have to heat the water to absorb the liquid and then set your metabolism to overdrive. The water will also fill your stomach more and leave less room for food while making you feel full enough.

Proper exercise is your ticket to more effective weight loss

If there is a secret to losing weight and keeping it away from the metabolism (your body's engine), it is that. Often surrounded by mystery, your metabolism is the speed at which your body burns fuel, and a healthy model is your best friend for burning fat and losing weight. Some people are blessed by the gods of a fast metabolism, but for most of us, we wish we could burn more fuel (calories) than we do right now.

It's worth it to understand the basics of metabolism because when it's properly conditioned and working properly (like a well-tuned car), it can significantly increase your efforts to lose weight. And the reverse is true, as a slow metabolism will hinder even the bravest efforts to lose weight.

Your metabolism is the key to losing weight.

Working to improve the "metabolic form" for better fat burning is the new way to lose weight and, above all, keep it off. When our hormones are balanced, our bodies burn the glucose produced by the food we eat for energy, and nothing or little is stored as excess in our body. And the reverse is also true, and when our metabolism is slow, it will store it as excess body fat, which is obviously how we are overweight.

For the past years, we have paid little attention to our exercise programs for metabolism health and weight loss focused only on what happened during a workout. But now things have changed, and the most important factor in an exercise program is what happens after it ends.

Of course, what you eat is important, but it's your exercise program that will help you determine where, when, and how the calories you eat are used. The low-intensity, long-lasting exercise that we thought was necessary for weight loss is not now considered the best type of exercise, as it is simply too low an intensity (degree of difficulty) to stimulate the fat-burning hormones.

Today, for faster weight loss, body composition (muscle / fat ratio) is what determines the health of your metabolism, and you can improve it with the adequate strength training exercise, which is the only type of exercise that will work directly. Muscles under load. It makes sense to get and keep your muscles healthy and toned since it is within the muscle cells that glucose is burned for energy.

Tones your muscles to lose weight quickly

Flabby and weak muscles have low energy needs and will not help you lose weight, which is why it is vital to recovering them in tonic conditions so that they can go to work to chew and burn that excess weight.

Your strength training program, performed at the correct intensity level, will ensure weight loss, as your metabolism will consume more fuel every minute of the day and night, even when you sleep or watch TV. This is what the subtle body you desire will return.

Get even faster weight loss results with a healthy eating plan that gives you the energy you need to train properly at a certain intensity. The wrong food choices (mainly processed foods) simply won't provide you with the fuel you need and instead reduce your energy levels. When you are not making a good food choice, you will not feel like being active, making weight loss much slower and more difficult.

You will have to become more active both with your exercise program and in your daily life, as this is what will rebuild your metabolic engine and burn more calories (stored body fat). Once done, you will be well on your way to winning the weight loss battle forever.

How to experience effective weight loss: learn more

Struggling with weight loss is not an easy task to accomplish, and this is further complicated by the various diet plans and exercise regimes that promise to offer effective results. As a result, most people who are trying to lose weight find the entire process frustrating and give up in half. In order to lose the extra pounds, you need to find a regimen that is reliable and effective, and there are several ways you can locate reliable and trustworthy products from the scam.

For starters, the chosen product must have the ability to absorb excess fat. There are cases when the body may not be able to achieve this goal. However, having excess fat could be the main reason why most people seem to add extra pounds at night. It is precisely for this reason that it is considered ideal to select a product with the ability to give the body the least amount of fat possible to obtain a better figure. If this is combined with a proper diet and regular exercise, it becomes easier to achieve that much-desired look.

Another important factor to consider before choosing any weight loss product is how it is marketed. It is important to select a product that guarantees weight loss and is clinically proven to do so. Consider that some diet or exercise is needed to accompany the product, as this is one of the main ways to determine if it is effective or not. In most cases, it is recommended to choose those products that have the ability to help achieve this without much effort. This is because this clearly shows that it is not only trustworthy but trustworthy in every sense of the word.

Consider how the product is rated by the average consumer and professionals. This is important since the production company can use a lot of advertising to market it, and yet it does not meet the required standards. Furthermore, knowing what other consumers have to say about the product, you can be sure that you will get the desired results with a higher level of efficiency. The best way to accomplish this is to do a little research on the Internet and read reviews. Also, discover the places where you can get genuine products to make sure you are safe.

More importantly, the products must be affordable. There are some products that are extremely expensive, and this only serves to increase the costs associated with weight loss. By selecting an inexpensive product, it becomes easier to follow the weight loss program.

Conditioning Your Mind For Effective Weight Loss

There is a wise saying that all things are created twice. The first creation is found in the realms of the mind. If you want to lose weight and get that slender figure, you have to condition your mind to think motivating thoughts that will soon manifest themselves as new habits for a healthy life.

Weight loss begins with a healthy lifestyle and the habit of eating the right types of food that will help you increase your weight loss effort. If you currently have an unhealthy lifestyle, moving to a more motivating and disciplined lifestyle can be quite challenging. The only way this can be accomplished is by strengthening your willpower and your mind so that you can easily overcome temptations.

The search for a healthier lifestyle begins with the formation of the right mental images and the strengthening of new beliefs that will ultimately lead to lasting changes in lifestyle.

If you are looking for ways to condition your mind to get into the right mindset, here are five simple steps.

Step 1: motivation

You must have the right motivation to be able to make mental changes in the new way of thinking and feeling. Start by finding the right reasons why you should want to lose weight and make it compelling. If you can find big enough reasons for the "why," you can always find the "how" to follow it.

Step 2: inspiring photos

You can start collecting photos that would inspire you to lose weight. Take nice pictures of bikini models or men in revealing outfits. Paste them in your diary, insert them in your wallet and view this image whenever you feel inclined to give up your weight loss program.

Step 3: statement

No, this does not mean that you should chant a strange mantra for half an hour a day. I am not a supporter of such canned affirmation approaches, but you have to get used to talking for yourself and convinced that there is no other way to live your life than with a thin and thin body.

Step 4: view

Spend several minutes daydreaming of yourself in your new sexy body, sailing on the sandy beaches, and getting the admired looks you desire. This can be a strong factor for starting to lose weight. Remember that what you see and think all day will move you to real life.

Step 5: reward yourself

A reward system is needed to help you stay on track and condition your sense to associate pleasant sensations with weight loss. Don't delay until you reach your final goal; reward yourself with each step.

Remember that the journey to a lean body is not a 100m race but a 1000 mile marathon that starts with one step. Get started, and the rest would be easy.

Weight loss: stay motivated

When losing weight, the biggest challenges can be motivating yourself. Weight loss is a long and slow process, and the results may not always be obvious. Therefore, finding ways to stay motivated is critical to your success. The surest way to fail at something is to quit smoking and lose motivation, and it will almost guarantee that you give up on your weight loss goals.

One of the vital things you can do to stay motivated is to set achievable goals. The goals you set must be realistic. Losing fifty pounds may be your goal, but it will probably be difficult to stay motivated when there are still forty-nine pounds left. Break it, decide that your goal is to lose five kilos in the following month. This is a realistic rate of weight loss and something you can really achieve.

Goal setting is rewarding when you reach your goal. Ideally, not with food, but within limits, it is also acceptable to enjoy junk food. The important thing is to be proud of what you have accomplished rather than worrying about how much you have left. No one likes to participate in an ungrateful task, so thanks to yourself.

There is no doubt that staying motivated can be a challenge. The main reason why most people fail to achieve their weight loss goals is simply to stop. It is essential that you stay motivated, or you will not have a chance to reach your weight loss goals.

One of the best ways to make your weight loss program more effective is through the use of supplements. One of the most effective weight loss supplements is the acai berry. An acai berry supplement will speed up your metabolism, provide you with the vitamins and minerals you need, and is an excellent source of antioxidants.

CHAPTER EIGHT

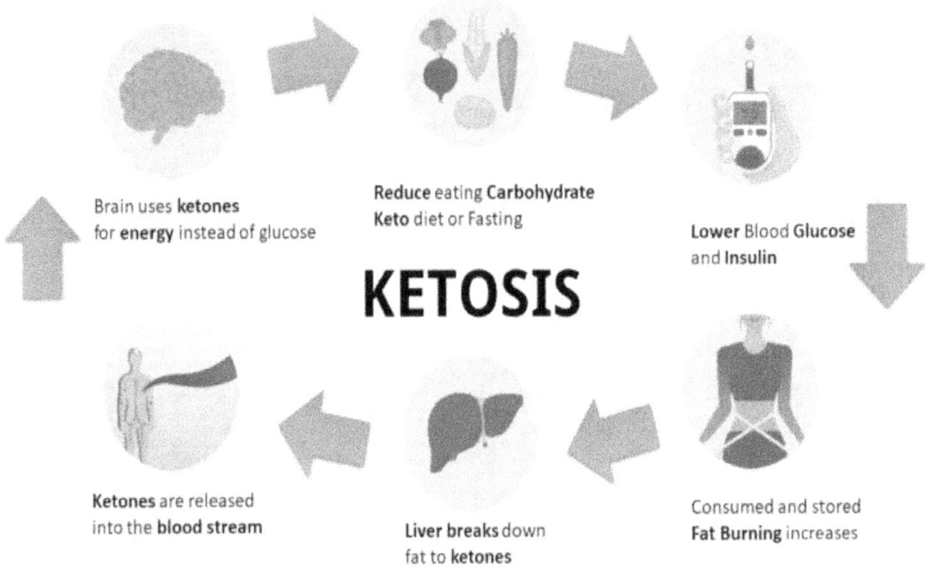

Howto get into ketosis on a keto diet

Important elements to increase your level of ketosis, classified from most important to least important:

Limit carbohydrates to 20 grams digestible per day or less, a strict diet low in carbohydrates or keto. Fiber should not be restricted, it could even be beneficial for the treatment of ketosis. Often, limiting carbohydrates to very low levels leads to ketosis. So, that may be all you need to do. But the rest of the list below will help you succeed.

Maintain a moderate protein intake. It is assumed that a keto diet is not a very high protein diet. You may want to eat about 1.5 g / kg of ideal body weight per day. That means about 100 grams of protein a day if you weigh 70 pounds (154 pounds).

Eating too much protein can prevent ketosis because the body converts excess protein into glucose. On the other hand, too little protein poses other health problems.

Eat enough fat to feel satisfied. A low-carb keto diet is usually a high-fat diet.53 This is the big difference between a keto diet and hunger, which also causes ketosis. A keto diet is sustainable, unlike famine.

When you starve, you are likely to feel tired and hungry and give up, but a ketogenic diet is sustainable and can make you feel good. Eat enough to feel satisfied and if you are constantly hungry, you should probably add more fat to your meals (like more butter, more olive oil, etc.).

Avoid itching when you are not hungry. Eat more than necessary, simply for pleasure and because there is food, it reduces acetosis and slows weight loss. Although the use of keto snacks minimizes the damage and that is good when you are hungry.

Add exercise: Adding any type of physical activity to a low carbohydrate content can moderately increase ketone levels. It can also help to slightly accelerate weight loss and the reversal of type 2 diabetes. Exercise is not necessary to fall into ketosis, but this can be useful.

Sleep: Get enough sleep, for most people at least seven hours per night on average, and control your stress. Sleep deprivation and stress hormones increase blood sugar levels, slow down ketosis and weight loss. In addition, they can make it more difficult to follow a keto diet and resist temptations. Therefore, even if controlling sleep and stress does not cause ketosis, it is worth thinking about.

Keto Rash

Following a ketogenic diet can sometimes cause an itchy red rash, commonly known as a keto rash. The medical term for keto rash is Prurigo pigmentosa. The keto rash is distinctive because it forms patterns similar to the networks of the skin. This usually affects the upper body. Researchers still do not know exactly why a ketogenic diet causes inflammation of the skin, but they think this rash may be related to ketosis. Several different treatments and lifestyle measures can relieve symptoms.

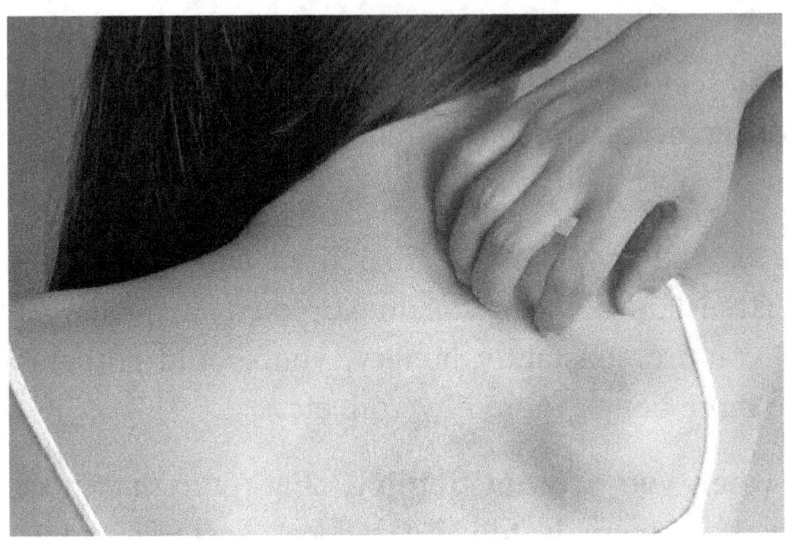

What is Keto Rash

Keto rash is a form of dermatitis that is itchy and uncomfortable. Ketogenic rash is a rare form of dermatitis or inflammation of the skin. It is an itchy, itchy rash that develops on the upper body.

A ketogenic diet is a possible cause of a keto rash. This diet is gaining popularity because ketosis offers a variety of potential health benefits, including weight loss. The keto diet is extremely low in carbohydrates but rich in protein and fat. When a person follows this diet pattern long enough, his body begins to break down body fat into fuel rather than carbohydrates. The body converts fat into ketone bodies.

A person has reached the state of ketosis when the body changes primary energy source for these ketone bodies. Most cases of keto-eruption have been reported in Japan, and in 2011, only 40 cases were reported in other countries. The reason may be that Western doctors are less aware of the disease.

<u>CAUSES</u>

The cause of the keto rash is unclear, but research suggests that being in ketosis may be a possible cause of the disease.

In addition to the keto diet, fasting and diabetes can result in a state of ketosis. Other possible causes or triggers of a keto rash are:

- hormonal changes that may occur during pregnancy and menstruation
- a complication of bariatric surgery
- skin friction

SYMPTOMS

The keto rash is in the form of raised, red, irritating papules. Redness of the skin or erythema may be more difficult to detect on dark skin.

Rashes are more common in the upper body and tend to affect:

- chest
- back
- neck

The ketogenic rash may resemble other skin conditions, such as confluent and reticulated papillomatosis, contact dermatitis, and some pharmacological reactions. However, it is possible to distinguish the keto rash by the networked pattern that remains in the skin when the red bumps begin to disappear. Over time, inflammation will continue to decrease, leaving a brownish discoloration of the skin.

TREATMENT

Moisturizing the area of the rash can relieve the symptoms.

There are several possible treatment options for a person with a rash.

For ketogenic ketosis eruptions, eating more carbohydrates will usually resolve the rash because the body will come out of it.

In diabetics, insulin can reduce keto rashs.

Research suggests that antibiotics, such as minocycline or tetracycline, may also treat the symptoms of the rash.

The friction between tight clothing and the skin can trigger the rash. Therefore, wearing loose clothing can also reduce it.

To relieve the symptoms, it is also helpful to follow the general treatment tips for good skin care, such as:

- avoid touching the rash whenever possible
- keep the nails short
- moisturize the area several times a day
- Avoid contact with irritants, such as wool or strong detergents.
- avoid hot or humid climates
- wash the skin gently and avoid excessive friction

The keto rash is rare. Researchers still do not fully understand the cause of the rash, but being in a state of ketosis may be a possible cause. Although there are similarities between keto rash and other skin conditions, this rash is distinctive due to the pattern of papule network.

People who develop a keto rash after a ketogenic diet or after fasting can treat it by increasing their carbohydrate intake. Doctors can also prescribe topical medications or oral antibiotics to help resolve the rash.

CONCLUSION

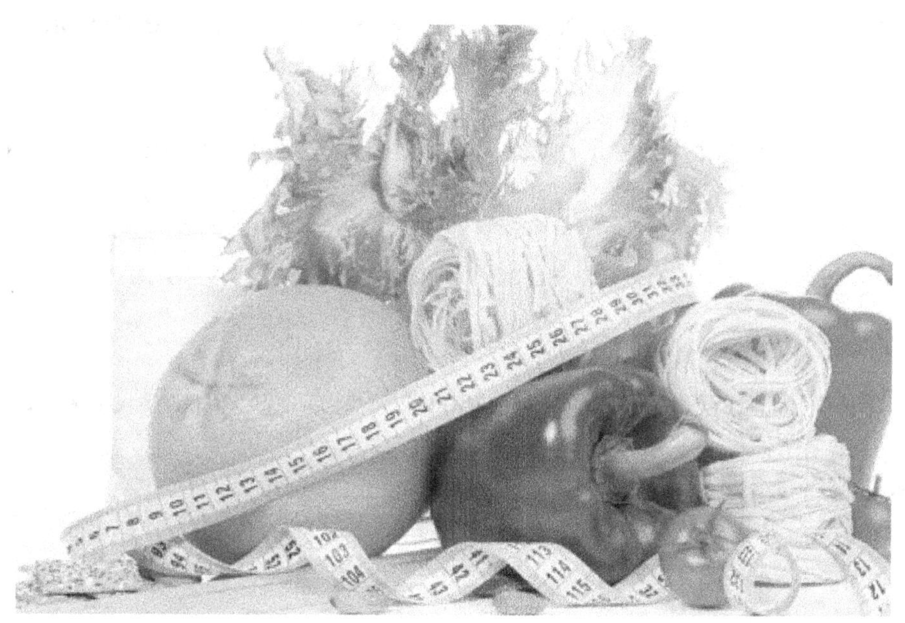

Frequently Asked Questions on Keto Diet

HOW DO I KNOW IF I HAVE KETOSIS?

Entering ketosis can take from 2 to 3 days to a few weeks, depending on your body's ability to adapt to burning fat as fuel. Once you enter ketosis, your body will naturally produce ketones, molecules that nourish your brain and body with fat, no carbohydrates.

You can usually tell if you have ketosis if you have consistent, long-lasting energy, better concentration, and reduced appetite. For definitive answers, test your ketone levels in the blood. You are in ketosis when your ketone levels are 0.8 (that is, millimoles per liter).

You can evaluate your levels with urine bars, blood bars or a blood drive. You can also assess the acetone levels in your breath using a breath analyzer. However, just follow the sensations of your body to find out if you have reached the optimal point of ketosis. Here are some signs that you are probably in ketosis:

Reducing Hunger: Ketones suppress hunger hormones and help you feel fuller longer.

Ketone breath: People often feel a metallic taste in their mouths because of high levels of ketone.

Weight loss: The keto diet burns fat, so if you lose weight, you are likely to suffer from ketosis.

Flu-like symptoms: At first, you may experience the symptoms of keto flu, such as headaches, chills, and dizziness.

DO I NEED TO CALCULATE THE MACROS AND HOW DOES IT COUNT?

Macros, or macronutrients, are the carbohydrates, fats and proteins that make up your food and help you create energy. It is not essential to count the macros in the keto diet, but it is a useful way to learn about your food and understand the needs of your body.

DO I NEED TO CALCULATE NET CARBOHYDRATES?

Even if you do not calculate macros, you must keep track of the net carbs, the carbohydrates that your body actually uses for energy. Calculating net carbs can help you stay ketosis and light up your food choices.

IS KETO DIET HEALTHY?

The ketogenic diet is healthy, effective and supported by science. When done correctly, it has been shown that the ketogenic diet helps to lose weight, creates more mitochondria in the brain, reduces inflammation and even fights metabolic syndrome diseases such as diabetes.

However, any diet can be good or bad for you, depending on what you put on your plate. If you stick to the foolproof diet roadmap, eliminate keto foods that make you feel weak and do not belong to a healthy diet, such as processed cheese and sugar-free soda.

WHAT ABOUT "DIRTY KETO?"

Dirty keto follows the same fat-rich and low-carb structure as the standard keto diet, but allows processed, packaged and fast foods. It is still possible to enter acetocetosis and burn fat when you are in a dirty keto, but this has serious drawbacks, such as inflammation and weight gain.

KETO SPIKE MY CHOLESTEROL?

Eating more saturated fats can increase your "good" HDL cholesterol, your total cholesterol and sometimes even your LDL cholesterol, and, contrary to popular belief, it's good if you eat high quality fats. Confused? This is what you need to know about diets high in cholesterol, saturated fat and carbohydrates.

DOES KETO DIET CAUSES DIABETES?

No, the keto does not cause diabetes. Several studies indicate that ketosis can help control diabetes by decreasing glucose intolerance and stabilizing blood sugar.

IS THE KETO DIET SUSTAINABLE LONG-TERM?

Yes and no. Some people eat without problems with the complete keto diet. Other people struggle with long-term carbohydrate restriction problems, such as insomnia and hormonal imbalances. If this is the case, try a cyto-cyclone keto-carb (cyclic ketosis), where you eat a moderate amount of carbohydrates one day a week, so that your body can enter and exit ketosis. It is an effective modification that helps many people avoid the dangers and risks of a keto diet.

WHAT ARE THE DIFFERENT TYPES OF KETONES?

There are three types of ketone bodies. They are:

Acetoacetate (AcAc): This is the first type of ketone that your body produces from fatty acids.

Beta-hydroxybutyric acid (BHB): Acetoacetate is converted to beta-hydroxybutyric acid. BHB is not really a ketone, due to its chemical structure, but it is still considered part of the ketone family because it works similarly to others. Fun fact: Brain octane oil, a purified form of MCT oil, is a precursor to BHB.

Acetone: byproduct of acetoacetate, acetone is the least abundant ketone in the blood. He leaves the body breathing or urine. The faster or you limit carbohydrates, the more you will produce more of each type.

HOW DO I KNOW IF I NEED MORE CARBONS?

Some people feel good when they eat too few carbohydrates for long periods. But if you have symptoms such as dry eyes, insomnia, tiredness and mood swings, your body may need more carbohydrates, especially if you are a woman, an athlete or face a lot of stress. (or all of the above).